SECTION 1
YOUR ACCIDENT

You have had a car accident. This is no fun; you did not plan for it and no one wants it. The choice is now yours: Be angry, feel wronged and upset or move forward. It has been shown that car accident patients who accept the fact that they were in a car accident and chose to move on with their lives do better than those who stay mad, upset and resentful.[1] Again – this is no fun, and you did not plan on this happening. The car accident experience is a stressful one and involves anger, frustration, worry and pain.[2] You are now faced with this next choice: Accept the accident and move on. Now it is time to move forward and work through the physical and emotional recovery after the car accident.

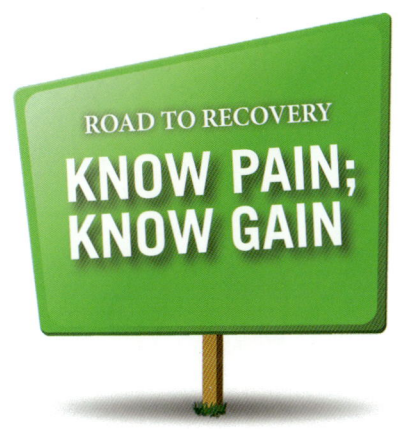

Thank you for taking the time to read this booklet. The booklet's goal is to explain what you will experience in the next few days, weeks and months after your accident. Studies have shown that patients who know more about what they can expect do better than those who do not.[2] This booklet will provide you with an understanding of how your nerves experience your neck pain and recovery after the accident.

> **You own both your neck and your pain. Your doctor, your physical therapist and your friends and family are there to help you, but you need to take control. With knowledge and effort, you will be able to do this; by doing this, you'll help yourself.**

SECTION 2
YOUR NERVOUS SYSTEM

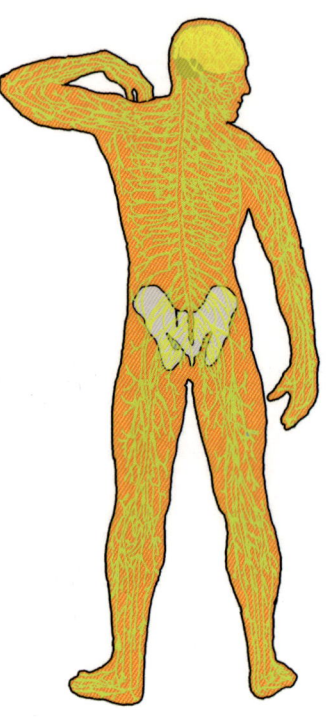

Your nervous system is a continuous structure with all the nerves in your feet, legs, back, upper back and arms connected and forming a network like a road system.[3] The main job of your nerves is to monitor your body and to inform you and your brain of anything going on in your body. Some nerves in your body work like an alarm system.[4]

Consider the example of when you step on a nail. You want to know about it so you can remove it, get a tetanus shot and not get an infection. The nerves in your foot need to send the message to your brain so that action can be taken. Nerves send messages by using electrical impulses.

At any given time, all nerves have a little bit of electricity running through them. This is normal and shows you are alive.[4,5]

When there is danger, such as a nail in the foot, the nerves increase electrical activity and

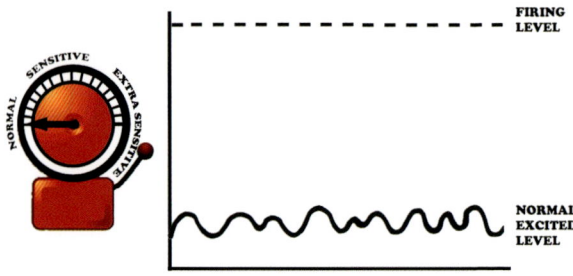

"wake up," sending a lot of danger messages to your spinal cord and ultimately to your brain. They let the brain know there is danger and action is required.[4-6]

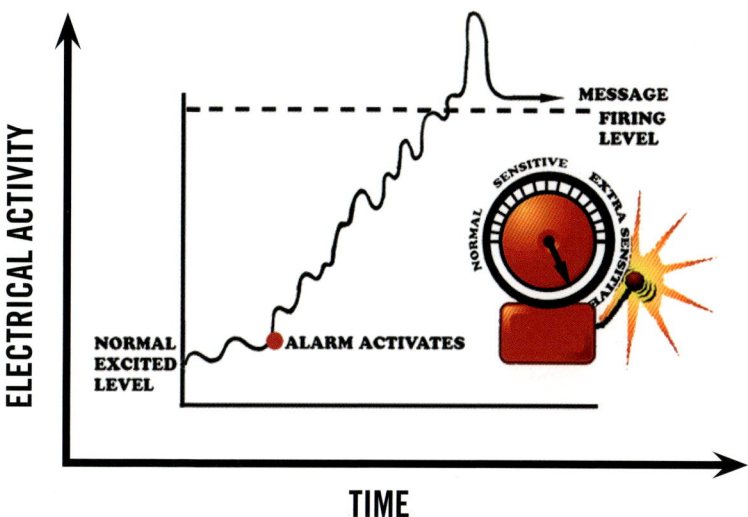

The brain's action may include walking funny, producing stress chemicals in your body or even using a choice word or two.

In this case, it is logical for the brain to produce pain in your foot so that you are alerted to the nail and you take action such as taking the nail out.

Once you take care of the danger, the nail in this case, it also makes sense for the alarm system to settle down and return to its normal resting level of activity ready for the next danger.[4-6] You will probably learn to avoid stepping on nails as well.

SECTION 3
YOUR NERVES AND YOUR NECK

When you hurt your neck in the accident, the same process as with the nail in the foot occurred.[7,8] When you developed neck pain, upper back pain and perhaps a headache, the nerves in your neck and upper back "woke up" alerting your brain to the danger in your neck and upper back. The nerves around the neck and upper back alerted the spinal cord, which in turn told the brain there is a problem in the neck and upper back.

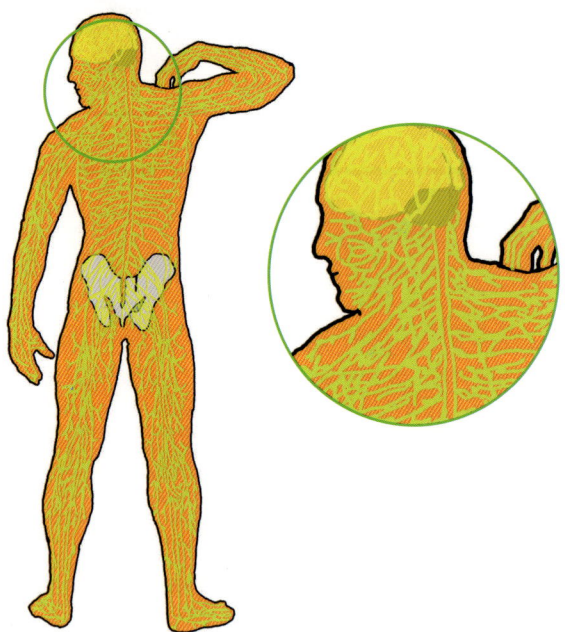

THE PAIN MAY CAUSE YOU TO DO THE FOLLOWING:
- ✓ See your family doctor
- ✓ See a physical therapist
- ✓ Have X-rays or an MRI
- ✓ Seek additional help

In essence, your nerves have done their job.

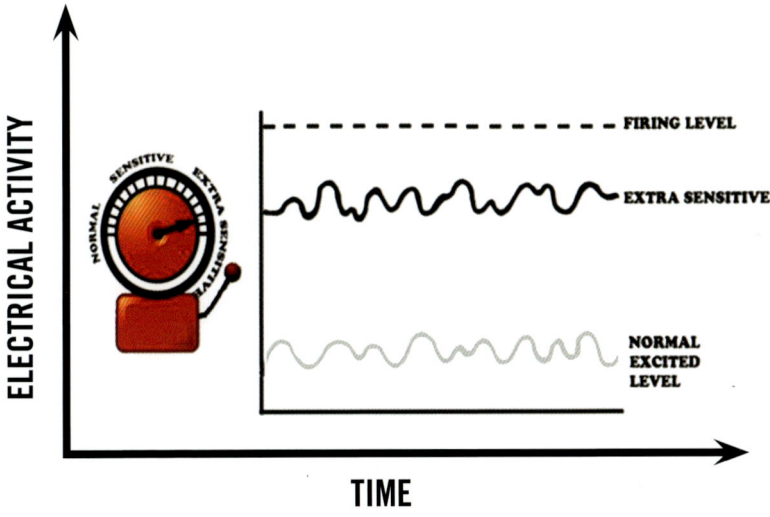

In some people, the nerves which "woke up" to alert you of the danger in your neck, upper back, head and perhaps your arm, calmed down very slowly and remained elevated and "buzzing."[7,9] In this state it does not take much activity such as sitting, reaching, bending or driving to get the nerves to fire off danger messages to the brain.

YOUR NERVES AND THEIR SENSORS

Inside your nerves there are various sensors also designed to protect and inform you of any changes in your life.[4,5,10]

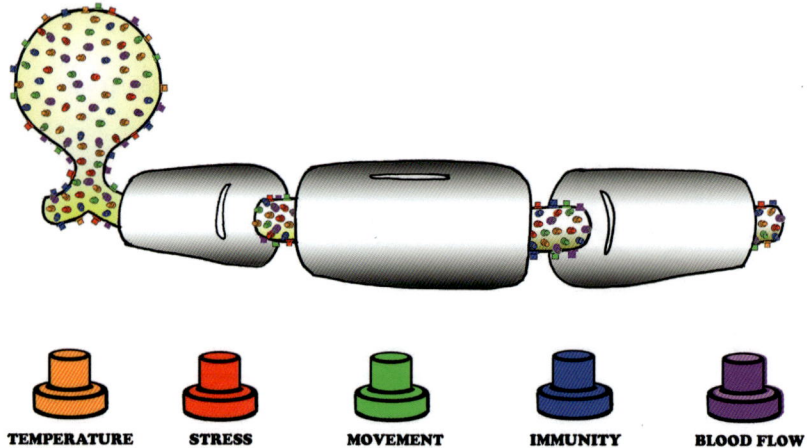

Various sensors have been identified, but the following may be of particular interest to you:

TEMPERATURE
There are sensors in nerves that tell you if there is a change in temperature. It is not uncommon to get sensitive to cold temperature and feel more aches and pains in the neck, upper back, head and arms when it gets cold out.[5,11]

STRESS
There are sensors in nerves which are sensitive to stress chemicals flowing in your blood. The more stressed, anxious, nervous or upset you are, the more you will experience a few more aches and pains. The more stress chemicals that run through your body, the more stress sensors are activated.[4,5,12]

BLOOD FLOW

There are sensors in your nerves that are sensitive to the amount of blood around your tissues. When blood flow slows down slightly, for example after sitting too long, these sensors "wake up" and make the nerves sensitive.[5,13]

MOVEMENT AND PRESSURE

There are sensors in your nerves which are sensitive to movement and pressure around them. For example, movement after the accident may activate a few more sensors and make the movement more sensitive for a little while.[4,5,14]

IMMUNITY

When you are sick with the flu for example, there are many immune molecules floating through your body helping you deal with the flu. This is the same following an injury. Recent research shows that when you are really worried and/or have an inflamed body part, you will have an immune response. Nerves have sensors telling them of the increased immune molecules, and the immune chemicals produced can make you ache.[14]

Key points about nerve sensors:

- ✓ **When you developed neck pain, your nerves increased their sensitivity to protect you.**
- ✓ **This is a normal response.**
- ✓ **These sensors are constantly updated based on your environment.**

Example: When you are in an accident such as yours, a little more anxiety is to be expected. In response to the slightly elevated stress chemicals in your blood, nerve sensors wake up, usually in and around the neck and upper back where the original injury is. Thus, you can "feel" your neck and upper back a little more. When stress levels ease, fewer sensors open and your sensitivity becomes less.

As mentioned before, in some people nerves are slow to calm down. Why is this? In some people there are so many issues surrounding the injured area that the brain decides it's best to keep the alarm system elevated. For example:

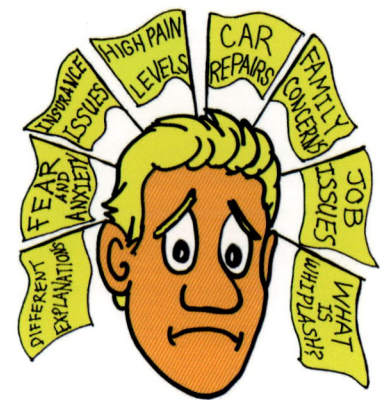

PAIN
Even though pain is a normal protective mechanism, the pain experience is stressful and simply no fun.[15] Shortly after the accident, it is quite normal to experience pain. This will lead to an elevated alarm system to protect you.

DIFFERENT EXPLANATIONS FOR YOUR PAIN
You can feel more stressed when you are not sure about what treatment option you should follow and have different explanations about what to expect.[16] Everyone has an opinion including family, friends and the Internet. All this uncertainty will leave the alarm system elevated for a while as you seek the answers.

FAMILY AND JOB
This accident has and surely will impact your family life and your job. This may include doctor and physical therapy visits, expensive tests, lost work time and frustration. In addition, there are concerns about being able to do your job, the future and money issues. This provides little incentive to your brain to turn the alarm system down. Add to this, concerns about getting the car fixed and even dealing with the insurance company.[17,18]

FEAR OF THE UNKNOWN
Unless you are a whiplash expert, there are many concerns and unknowns. The uncertainty is usually accompanied by some anxiety or fear. This is quite common, but it has been shown that fear of injury, re-injury, and fear of exercise or movement is likely to keep the alarm system turned on rather than off.[19]

YOUR NERVOUS SYSTEM'S NEIGHBORS WAKE UP

When your nerves in your neck "wake up," there are usually some interested neighbors. Remember that your nervous system is connected (Section 2). Consider the nervous system as an alarm system. If the alarm in your house goes off, it probably wakes the neighbors right next to you. They are curious and concerned about you. If the alarm keeps going, some neighbors down the street may wake up. Nerves work the same way. Since your neck, upper back and even arm's alarm systems have been awakened, it is common for the neighboring tissues such as the lower back and head to be awakened.[20] It is not uncommon to experience some sensitivity in your lower back, upper back and neighboring areas after the accident.

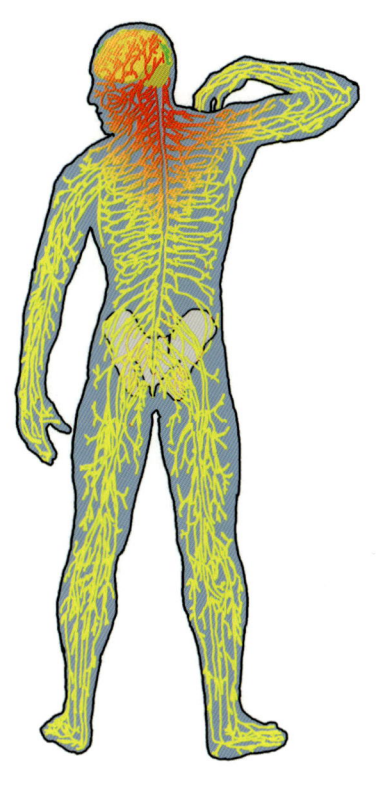

> The important issue for you to understand is that your pain may not only be due to the original accident, but also to the increased sensitivity of the nerves in the region and neighboring areas.

SECTION 4
YOUR ACCIDENT AND YOUR SPINAL NERVES

The term "whiplash" is the mechanism where by your neck, due to the accident, undergoes sudden movement.[1] Although the muscles and joints of our necks are designed for movement, they do not like sudden movement. In a car accident, the sudden movement causes some joints to be sprained,

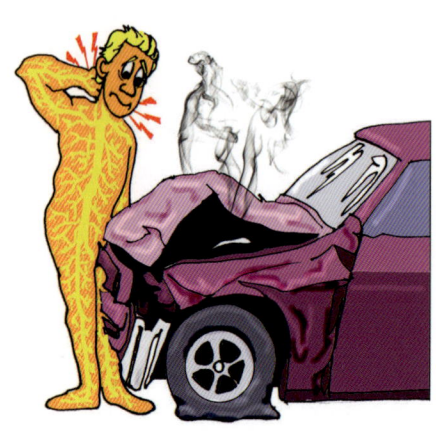

similar to an ankle sprain.[21] This in turn leads to inflammation and swelling. Every day after the accident, these joints and muscles will undergo a healing process. Every day is better. They eventually heal in a matter of weeks. These joints and muscles; however, are all surrounded by these sensitive nerves we have been discussing. A large part of your recovery is calming the nerves to coincide with the healing of the tissues.

To perform at their best, your nerves need three things: **space, movement and blood.**

❶ SPACE
As your nerves travel through your body, they run through little holes through and around muscles and many other tissues. If these spaces are closed down due to swelling and inflammation, the nerve will become sensitive and irritated. Arm pain along with neck pain is an example of this happening. With the healing of the tissues, medication, gentle early movement and time, these spaces open giving the nerve back its space and easing pain.

❷ MOVEMENT

Nerves are designed to slide and glide. When nerves get irritated, it takes away some of the ability of the nerve to slide. This limits your movement which may activate nerve sensors making them more sensitive. Early, gentle and frequent movement of the neck, upper back, arms and body will all allow the nerves to slide and glide more easily, thus easing pain.

❸ BLOOD

About 25% of all the blood and oxygen in your body is used by your nerves; nerves thrive on blood. When nerve movements are limited, it may cause some discomfort as the nerve may not have enough blood around it. Nerves that have lots of blood and oxygen around them calm down, which is why it is a good thing to do aerobic exercise such as brisk walking as part of your recovery plan.

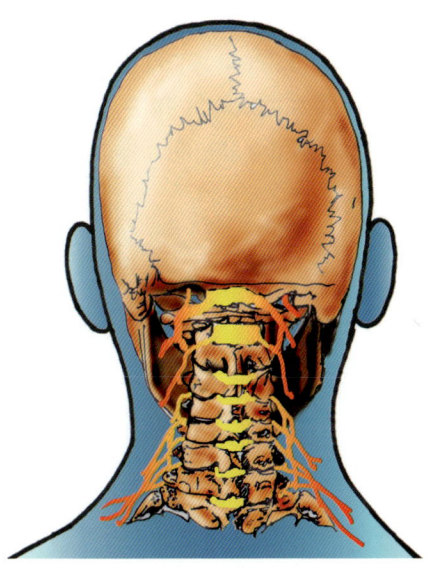

NOW FOR THE IMPORTANT PART:

As soon as the accident is over, each day brings healing. The body's healing process, use of medication and gentle, frequent movement will allow the joints to move and recover. This is one part of the recovery process.

Your nerves, even though they now have enough space and are more able to slide and glide and probably happy about some blood and oxygen, will still be sensitive. If you consider that nerves need space, movement and blood, it is a good thing to move after the accident. The fact that your nerves are still somewhat sensitive after the accident is expected and explained in this booklet.

> **With all the irritation, the nerve is still in "alarm mode." With the healing, medication and gentle movement opening the space, attention should now focus on calming the nerves down.**

YOUR ACCIDENT, MEDICAL EXPERIENCE AND YOUR NERVES

It is also important for you to understand that your accident and subsequent hospital experience can be somewhat stressful and may in the short term make your nerves even more sensitive as follows:

EMERGENCY CARE AT THE ACCIDENT SITE

Each person in a car accident has a different experience regarding the care they receive at the accident site. In some cases people are just shook up, seemingly fine and prefer to see their family doctor in a few days or see how they feel in a few days before seeking medical help. In other cases, patients are examined at the accident site by emergency personnel and taken to the emergency department. This busy, noisy environment and ultimate transport to the hospital is stressful. Anxiety, fear of the unknown and stress will undoubtedly keep your nerves "awake." This is normal.[22,23]

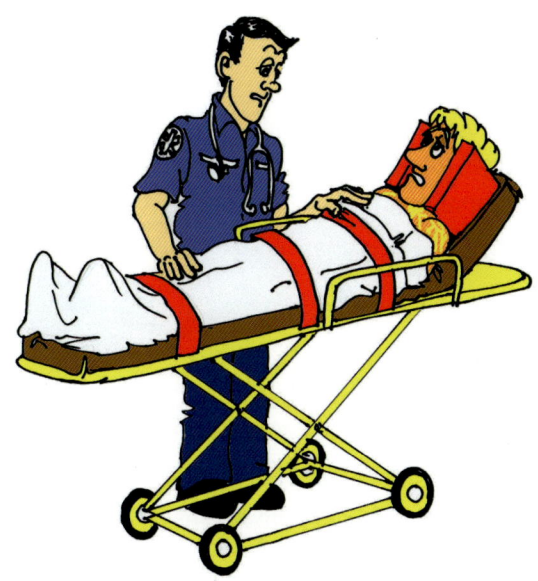

HOSPITAL PROCEDURES

As you deal with the accident and medical care, you need to deal with hospital procedures such as check in, various hospital personnel, tests and questions. Unless you're an experienced hospital goer, these procedures may also add to your anxiety and nerve sensitivity.[24]

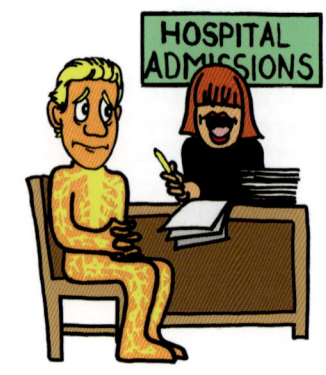

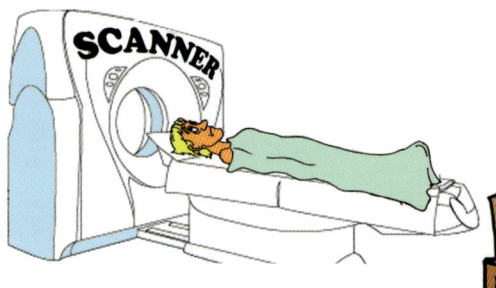

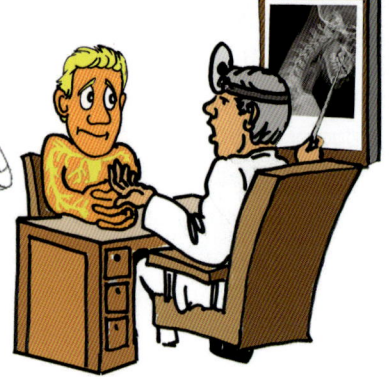

MEDICAL CONSULTATION

Following the accident, you will undoubtedly see your family physician for a follow-up. Usually, this is all that is needed so your physician can track your progress. In some cases you may be referred to see a specialist. All of these visits are stressful and may even add some anxiety.

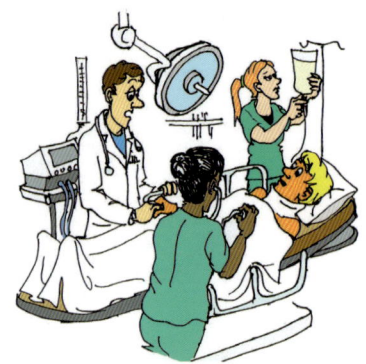

> The important issue for you to understand is that your pain may not only be due to the original accident, but also to the increased sensitivity of the nerves in the region and neighboring areas.

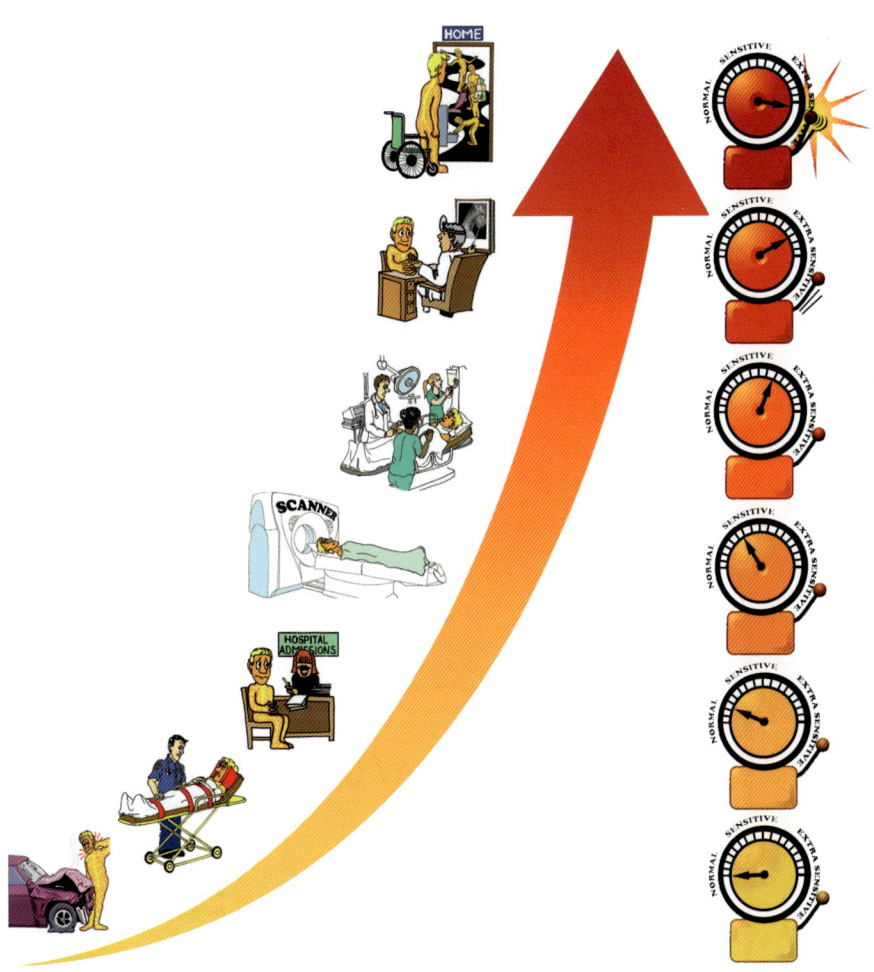

Apart from your nerves having "awakened" due to the accident, they will likely be very reactive to the overall hospital and medical treatment experience. Each part of this process may add to a few more alarm signals from the nerves.

SECTION 5
YOUR NERVES WILL CALM DOWN

How do you calm nerves down, turn the alarm system down and treat pain? There are basically three things you can do to help yourself:

❶ KNOWLEDGE

The good news is you are already getting started. Research has shown that the more you understand about pain and how pain works, the better you will do.[25-27] As you read this booklet and gain an increased understanding of the sensitivity of your nerves as part of your pain experience, what you learn actually calms your nerves down by turning down the alarm system.[15,28]

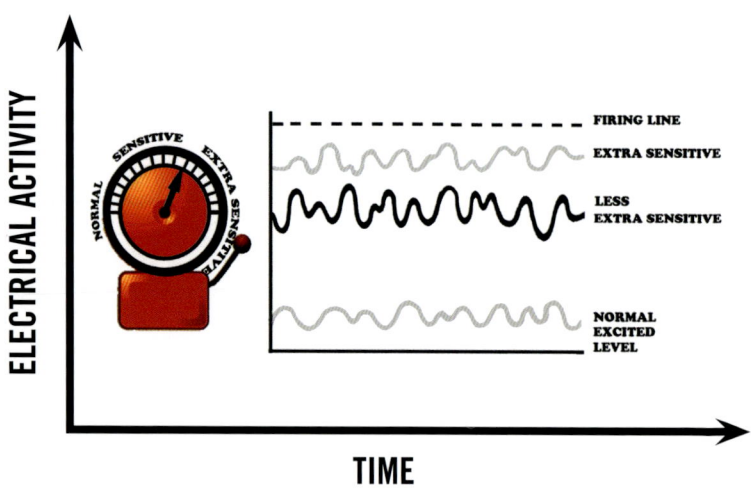

❷ MOVEMENT

Nerves love blood.[5,29] Scientists have shown that when we pump blood and oxygen around nerves, they actually calm down.[30] Exercise that promotes blood flow, such as aerobic exercise like brisk walking will help calm your nerves down over time.

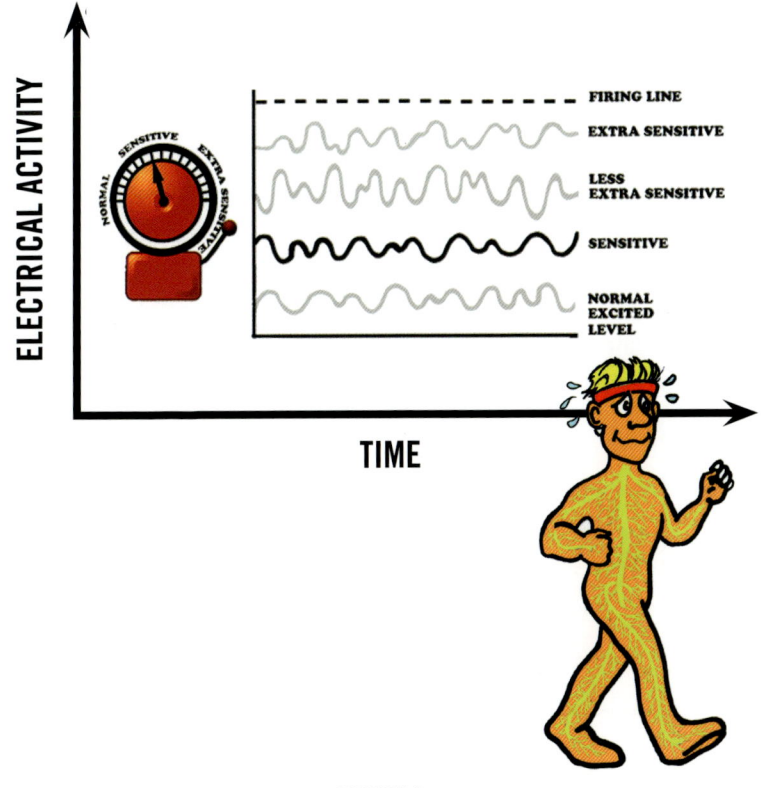

Immediately after the accident, start walking. Leg and trunk movements, without putting undue stress on the neck, are a great way to get blood and oxygen flowing through your body. The walking will also aid in helping you calm your nerves. In addition, begin gently moving your neck from side to side as well as up and down. Remember – hurt does not equal harm.

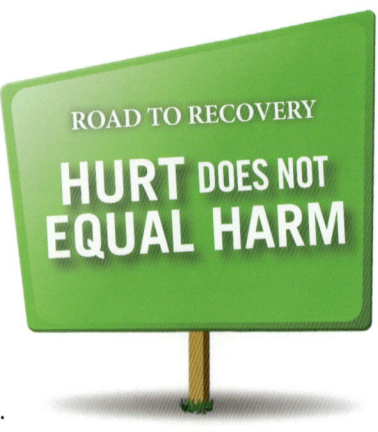

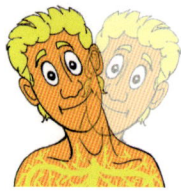 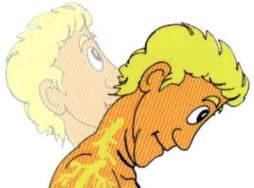 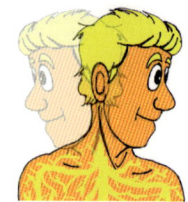

❸ MEDICATION

There are medications designed to calm nerves down.[31] Your doctor may discuss this with you. You may even be taking them now. Ideally over time, you will be able to decrease the need for these medications as you recover. The pain you experience is affected by very powerful chemicals in the brain. Although many people can name five pain medications you can buy over the counter, few know the potent chemicals your brain produces that work like pain medication. The world's most sophisticated and powerful medicine cabinet is located in your brain.[4,32] The brain uses chemicals such as endorphins, enkephalins, opioids and serotonin to help us ease pain.

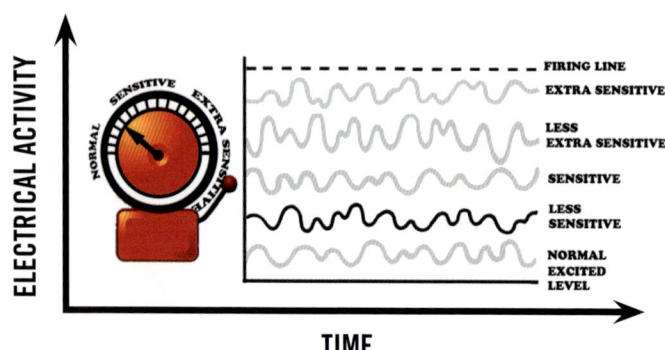

SECTION 5

WET BRAIN

A wet brain is the description of a brain with a faucet turned open and flushing pain medication down the spinal cord to dampen incoming danger messages. When you stub your toe, you may experience a lot of pain for a short while; the toe hurts less a few seconds later. In this case, the brain uses these chemicals to ease the pain experience. These drugs are also potent in survival stories and stories where people have extensive injuries yet experience little to no pain.[4]

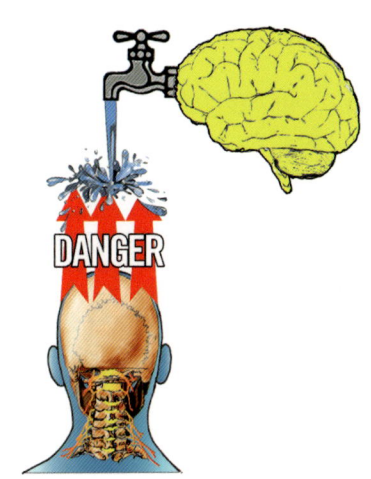

DRY BRAIN

A dry brain is the opposite. In this scenario, the faucet is closed. The longer you experience pain, the brain produces less of the pain medication. Although it seems contrary, it is a survival strategy by your brain. Remember that your brain is getting more worried about your neck, upper back and arm. Because of this, it makes sense to the brain to dry up or close the tap and stop the medicine altering the pain experience.[4]

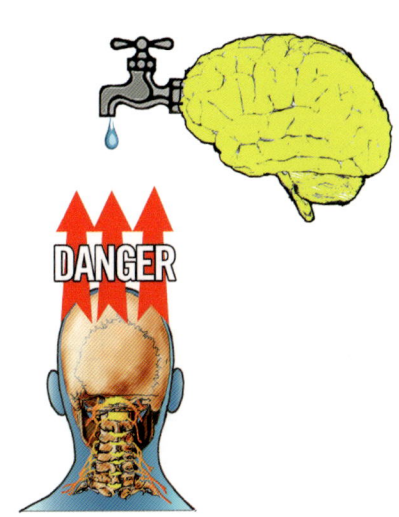

KNOWLEDGE IS MEDICINE.

The more you know about your pain, accident and nerves, the more likely your brain will protect you and develop a wet brain to help turn the alarm system down.

SECTION 6
YOUR RECOVERY AFTER THE ACCIDENT

- ✓ Your experiences related to your neck and upper back are normal and can be explained.

- ✓ Your experiences are stressful and have caused your nerves, your alarm system, to wake up. This is a normal process.

- ✓ Your pain is real. The healing, medicine and gentle movement is designed to give the nerve back some space, but some of the pain is due to increased nerve sensitivity.[33]

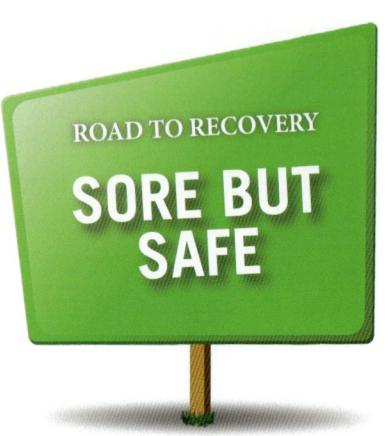

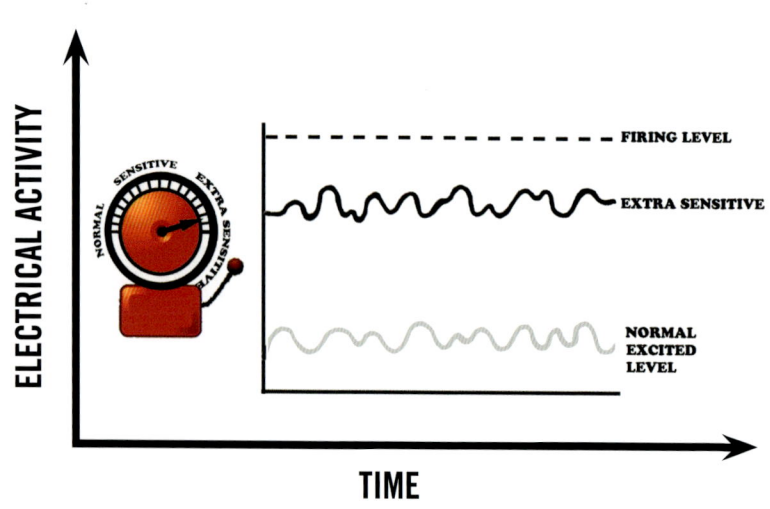

- ✓ Your alarm system is sophisticated. It is unlikely your alarm system will completely turn off immediately, but rather remember the experience and over time turn down.

- ✓ Your alarm system will steadily be turned down. As your neck heals, you work on recovery and gain increased understanding of your neck and its recovery, the nerve sensitivity will decrease over weeks and months.

- ✓ Your recovery will have ups and downs, and some flare ups, which is expected. The flare ups are not due to harm, but rather due to sensitivity.[4]

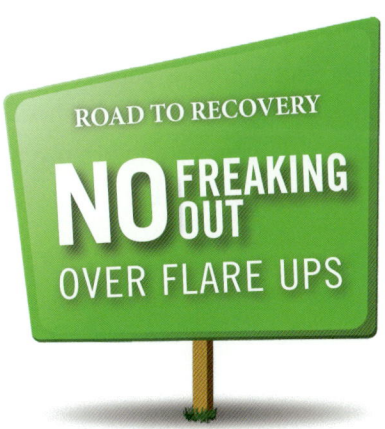

- ✓ Your nerves are barometers for the stresses of life. The more stressed you are, the more neck, upper back and possibly arm pain you may experience. The calmer you are, the less pain you will experience.

✓ Your recovery requires movement after the accident.[33] Your doctor and physical therapist will give you advice on movement after the accident. As you heal and recover, work on increasing your exercises, movement and walking program. Movement that gets blood and oxygen flowing around your nerves will help calm your nerves down as well as benefit your lungs and general health.[30]

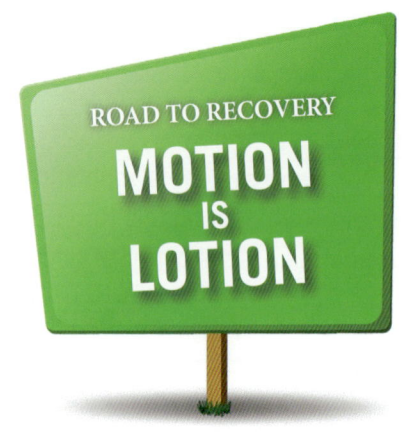

✓ Your medication after the accident will help calm down the alarm system. Medication also helps the brain to produce more of its own pain medication, thus creating a wet brain.

✓ Your doctor, his or her staff and your physical therapist can help answer any questions you may have. As you should realize by now, the more confused, nervous or uncertain you are, the more extra sensitive the alarm system will be.

✓ In 2-3 weeks you may have a follow up visit with your doctor. As time goes on, these post-accident visits will spread out to coincide with your recovery.

CONCLUSION

When you hurt your neck your nerves "woke up" to protect you. The healing, medication and gentle frequent movement will help give the nerve back some much needed space, movement and blood. Your nerves are extra sensitive. The more you know about how your nerves work and what causes their sensitivity, the better you will be. Knowledge, gentle movement and realistic goals will help your nerves to calm down over time, leading to a successful recovery from your car accident.

QUESTIONS FOR YOUR DOCTOR OR THERAPIST

Knowledge is power. The more you know about your accident and its affect on your nerves, the better you will be. Use this page to list questions you want to ask your doctor or physical therapist:

SCIENTIFIC SUPPORT FOR YOUR RECOVERY

1. Spitzer WO, Skovron ML, Salmi LR, et al. Scientific monograph of the Quebec Task Force on Whiplash-Associated Disorders: redefining "whiplash" and its management. Spine. Apr 15 1995;20(8 Suppl):1S-73S.

2. Van Oosterwijck J, Nijs J, Meeus M, et al. Pain neurophysiology education improves cognitions, pain thresholds, and movement performance in people with chronic whiplash: A pilot study. J Rehabil Res Dev. 2011;48(1):EPub ahead of print.

3. Louw A, Mintken P, Puentedura L. Neuophysiologic Effects of Neural Mobilization Maneuvers. In: Fernandez-De_Las_Penas C, Arendt-Nielsen L, Gerwin RD, eds. Tension-type and Cervicogenic Headache. Boston: Jones and Bartlett; 2009:231-245.

4. Butler D, Moseley G. Explain Pain. Adelaide: Noigroup; 2003.

5. Butler D. The Sensitive Norvous System. Adelaide: Noigroup Publications; 2000.

6. Louw A, Puentedura EL, Mintken P. Use of an abbreviated neuroscience education approach in the treatment of chronic low back pain: a case report. Physiotherapy theory and practice. Jan 2012;28(1):50-62.

7. Jull G, Sterling M, Kenardy J, Beller E. Does the presence of sensory hypersensitivity influence outcomes of physical rehabilitation for chronic whiplash?--A preliminary RCT. Pain. May 2007;129(1-2):28-34.

8. Louw A. Management of the whiplash patient. In: S.B. B, Manske R, eds. Clinical Orthopaedic Rehabilitation. 3rd Edition ed. Philadelphia, PA: Elsevier; 2011.

9. Sterling M, Treleaven J, Jull G. Responses to a clinical test of mechanical provocation of nerve tissue in whiplash associated disorder. Man Ther. May 2002;7(2):89-94.

10. Devor M. The pathophysiology and anatomy of damaged nerve. In: Wall PD, Melzack R, eds. Textbook of Pain. Edinburgh: Churchill Livingstone; 1984:49-64.

11. Fournier E, Viala K, Gervais H, et al. Cold extends electromyography distinction between ion channel mutations causing myotonia. Ann Neurol. Sep 2006;60(3):356-365.

12. Madden KS. Catecholamines, sympathetic innervation and immunity. Brain Behav Immun. 2003;17(S1):5-10.

13. Igarashi T, Yabuki S, Kikuchi S, Myers RR. Effect of acute nerve root compression on endoneurial fluid pressure and blood flow in rat dorsal root ganglia. J Orthop Res. Mar 2005;23(2):420-424.

14. Milligan ED, Twining C, Chacur M, et al. Spinal glia and proinflammatory cytokines mediate mirror-image neuropathic pain in rats. J Neurosci. Feb 1 2003;23(3):1026-1040.

15. Moseley GL. A pain neuromatrix approach to patients with chronic pain. Man Ther. Aug 2003;8(3):130-140.

16. Louw A, Butler DS. Chronic Pain. In: S.B. B, Manske R, eds. Clinical Orthopaedic Rehabilitation. 3rd Edition ed. Philadelphia, PA: Elsevier; 2011.